FOLLOWING THE FOOTSTEPS OF REAL HEALING

PREFACE

What is described in this book is an updated version of ancient medicine knowledge. For centuries, people have benefited from some alternative treatments other than modern medicine. This book is full of information that will help to protect our health and to improve its quality by supporting modern medicine.

What is the Immune System ?

The immune system must be healthy; this is very important. If the immune system is not strengthened, there will be no health. It is the immune system that treats human disease. The main disease is malnutrition and lifestyle. People have never consumed so many additives and so many, abundant and varied foods in any period of history. For this reason, the liver of people has turned into garbage in this century. According to the "Chronic Diseases Report", the number of patients is constantly increasing. Being sick is one's own fault. Because his body has such an excellent Immune System that protects him from diseases, it is necessary to "struggle" to destroy this mechanism.

What should we eat to strengthen the immune system?

The importance of strengthening the immune system once again came to the agenda in the last days when infections increased. So what are immune-boosting supplements ? Onions, garlic, natural honey, natural molasses, lemon, ginger, turmeric, pollen, natural kefir and natural yogurt, sage, unroasted nuts, fish (especially omega 3 should be noted), and finally natural fruit and vegetable strengthen immunity. There might be no need for supplement vitamins for immunity. Someone who is already naturally fed does not need vitamins.

 The most important basis of natural nutrition technique is nutrition according to the temperament. Nutrition according to blood groups is the basis of this technique and makes the human body suitable for the temperament of creation. For this reason, the body fed by this technique will always have the highest level of resistance to diseases. Therefore, the best method of protection against illnesses is this nutrition technique in addition to social distance and cleaning methods. In this book, we will consider the main ingredients of this nutrition technique one by one. With this nutrition technique, which has benefited many people, we hope that all of our readers will contribute to their health. LET'S BEGIN !

Temperaments/Blood Groups

In the times before blood groups were determined as determined by today's medicine, physicians divided people into groups according to their temperaments and tried to treat people's diseases according to those temperaments. Physicians have determined that there are different temperaments in humans as well as in different types of goods and fruits. They found that the same distinction exists in animals. Not only that, they also classified food according to temperament. In the first book of the famous El-Kânûn Fi't- Tıbb (Law in Medicine) of Ibn-i Sînâ, who was the authority in medicine, the third part is devoted to these temperaments.

While writing these nutrition articles according to the blood group, I will especially benefit from the temperaments section of Ibn-i Sina's famous book El-Kânûn Fi't- Tıbb (Law in Medicine). I will also benefit from the knowledge of deceased Doctor Aidin SALIH [1], other researcher-authors (Mehmet Ali Bulut [2]).

The human digestion process is very important. "A person's morality is directly related to the food he eats and digestion," says Dr. Aidin Salih [1]. Of course, it is not possible to divide people into four groups in terms of digestion process according to their blood. The blood type determined to date is around 125,000. There are basically four blood groups. These are also divided into two as (Rh +) and (Rh -). In addition, if we add that each blood group is actually in binary pairs, namely AA-A0, BB-B0, AB and 00, we can talk about 12 different blood groups with the Rh factor.

Digestion in Blood Groups

Extensive analysis made today shows that; even in the same blood group, different sensitivities can be seen in the digestion process. The digestion process is related to human intestinal flora. Food digestion may differ from person to person. Despite such diversity, it is still possible to categorize foods according to certain blood groups and then consume consumption accordingly. Ancient physicians separated people according to their temperament and applied treatments accordingly. According to them, the number of basic temperaments is four: Phlegmatic temperament, Sanguine temperament, Choleric temperament, Melancholic temperament.

According to the ancient doctors, nobody is from this or that temperament. Everyone is in a structure consisting of a certain mixture of these above-mentioned temperaments. Ancient physicians stated that there are 64 kinds of basic temperaments. Based on temperaments, while bread to someone with the same blood group is beneficial, it may not be beneficial to the other. Therefore, if the person determines what is working or not for his body and becomes a doctor for himself by this way , he will do a healthy job. Attention to this point : If a person experiences heartburn and indigestion after eating any kind of food, then he or she shall avoid that food. Because indigestion is the head of all diseases. This is the best remedy! The main factor that harms the body is food that cannot be digested.

Now I will give you a few examples based on my own eating and drinking experiences. I can easily say that it is possible to correct blood pressure, reflux, migraine, triglyceride, cholesterol, headache, gastrointestinal diseases by good chewing, changing the wrong lifestyle, paying attention to the method of eating and drinking according to the blood group. I am from O blood group. If I eat white bread and dairy products or a food made from white flour, itching immediately recurs, such as eczema. Because the group 0 must eat exact wheat or rye.

If someone from blood type A eats the veal 2 or 3 times on the same day, gets sick. Or he/she can not fully digest. That person's bile does not melt the beef. He/she should eat meat at most one day a week. For example: One day, a friend of 0 blood group said 1 and a half portions of pita bread. There is no problem in meat for group 0. But the dough made from white flour is a nuisance for the 0 group. Even though I warned, he ate. I later learned that he had eaten some of the pita of another friend next to him. So, more than 2 servings. Days later he called me. "I dealt with hemorrhoids for a full week," he said.

I want to say that; in my family circle and among my relatives and close friends, I observed the accuracy of this food classification. Nutrition according to the blood group is not a subject that will end with just one article. Issues such as which blood group is prone to cancer, and which blood group will have more tooth decay,etc... will be written by taking advantage of the opinions of deceased Doctor Aidin Salih [1] who is the authority on these issues and of other authors (M.Ali Bulut [2]).

<u>**Protecting ' Temperament Properties' and ' Inner Knowledge'.**</u>

It is possible to see this issue in children, because they have the most obvious temperament characteristics. If meat, rice, chicken and bulgur pilaf are offered to 4 children with different blood groups; group A prefers chicken pilaf or bulgur (cracked wheat) pilaf, does not want pilaf with meat; group O prefers meat pilaf or chicken pilaf, does not want bulgur (cracked wheat) pilaf; group B prefers pilaf with meat and does not want chicken pilaf.

In times when transportation was not as fast as it is today, people were fed in accordance with the temperament because they had temperament characteristics compatible with the region they live in and did not have such an excessive and mixed eating habits, and they did not use synthetic foods. Today, we need the concept of blood group due to the thousands of kinds of mixed foods that reach our regions from all over the world with the development of transportation. As a matter of fact, those who are fed according to the blood group relax after a while and start to get rid of their excess weight. The reason for this is that the foods suitable for the blood group are easily digested and the amount of metabolic waste is minimized. When the person gets rid of the waste materials that accumulate in his body and cause illness and when the body regains the internal information, he does not need the concept of blood group.

In addition, if the person who is based on the ancient knowledge of nutrition and does not get eager to eat, and is satisfied with about 400 grams of food he/she needs daily, foods will not bother him/her even if they do not match his/her blood group. It is a serious mistake if a wide variety of nutrients that do not match the enzymes necessary for digestion are consumed together and are also consumed in large quantities, and in addition, foods that do not fit the blood group are eaten. And, as it repeats, it slowly takes the person towards the disease.

In summary, in response to the above issues, a healthy person can eat everything that Allah makes halal and wants, regardless of the blood type, within the limits recommended by the Messenger of Allah. The nutrition of the patients according to the blood group facilitates the immune system's struggle to restore health.

We continue our nutrition articles according to blood groups. Diseases are also linked to the blood group. In that case, a person has a predisposition to certain diseases, but there is no such thing as a certain disease. An illness can only occur if there is a disease, and it also occurs if the person makes mistakes. We all know that, otherwise it will not appear. It is possible to recognize diseases immediately by looking at the blood group. When a doctor learns the patient's blood type and look at his diet, he will understand the situation. And doctors also may ask, "What is the blood group? Has breast milk taken in childhood? What oils and chemicals does that person use? ". After receiving the answers to these questions, the situation becomes more obvious.

Hemoglobin value is very important according to blood groups. Hemoglobin is the most important substance of red blood cells in the blood, consisting of iron, nitrogen, oxygen, hydrogen, coal and sulfur, providing oxygen and carbon gas transmission between the lungs and the eyes. Low hemoglobin levels usually indicate that a person has anemia. The high hemoglobin value causes the body to make too much red blood cells and make the blood thicker than normal. This can lead to clots, heart attacks, brain bleeding, and strokes. It may also lead to polycythemia vera (a blood disorder where your bone marrow forms too many red blood cells).

Hemoglobin Value According to Blood Groups

According to Dr. Aidin SALIH [1], it is an excellent condition that hemoglobin is 10 in those with blood group A. No higher blood is needed for group A. It is perfect for hemoglobin to be 13 in blood group O, 13-15 in blood group B, 13 in blood group AB, just like blood group O. When hemoglobin is 15 (except B), it can be said that this is not good. Then it is necessary to reduce blood. Having hemoglobin more than 15 is very dangerous. Then it is necessary to reduce the blood immediately because in this case dangers such as heart attack and brain hemorrhage increase.

NUTRITION ACCORDING TO BLOOD GROUPS

* (Blood Group O)

Dr. Aidin SALIH [1] says: "The cause of indigestion is unique, and that is to eat food that is not suitable for nature. Because eating unfit for nature is a disease." For example, for those with a blood group of O or A, drinking milk is a complete grind. Then they will have indigestion. Or they get diarrhea that is the best case. Since blood group B and O are carnivorous, they need to eat meat. Then his teeth will be perfect. But if a person with a blood group of O does not consume meat , or if he has been fed pastries since he was little, he remains toothless. Teeth rot, melt and disappear.

In this case, unused stomach acid rises to the ears and burns all the teeth, melts the palate, and also causes angina and chronic pharyngitis. But the meat-eating blood group O, B, and AB have good teeth. If those with a blood group of O are obliged to eat rice, wheat and wheat products, they should eat them fatty. (Olive oil, butter and animal fat) If they do this, their stomach will be comfortable. They should definitely consume the date by dipping it in olive oil. When those who have blood group O leave wheat and dairy products, their stomachs return to normal. They can eat yogurt. But they need to drink milk when they get older . Because stomach acid decreases. But they shouldn't drink it every day when they get older. If they drink, they start with restlessness, then calcification and other ailments.

Only blood group 0 can be pure blood group. If there is a blood group of 0 among children, the mother or father will definitely have a blood group of 0. If the parent does not carry 0, the child cannot carry 0. Although the blood type of the mother and father is A, the blood type of the child can be 0. This means that both parents carry 0. Those with a blood group of 0 generally remain toothless and palate. Because the characteristic of those with 0 blood type is that their upper palate is short and their fingers are long.

M.Ali Bulut [2] says in his book: "I see the digestive system of those with zero blood type as vehicles powered by diesel engines. They can eat every kind of meat. Bread is inconvenient." In fact, the person whose blood type is zero should eat those made from whole wheat or rye flour, even if they eat cookies. The main diseases encountered by people with zero blood group are: Heartburn, gastritis, chronic pharyngitis, reflux, ulcerative enteritis, stomach ulcer, calcification, sputum production, kidney and gallstone formation, skin cancer, larynx cancer and elephant disease. They always complain of heartburn. They love to complain. They especially experience heartburn in the evening. Because they can digest in the morning and not in the evening. Every meal eaten with bread in the evening, especially if meatless, causes heartburn. Its name is reflux. It occurs especially if it is eaten late.

Especially, if they drink black tea with sugar and dark, there will be bloating. They should drink tea with honey, unroasted nuts or unrefined sugar. Gastric acid of blood group zero is too much. There is no problem with stomach acid. The problem is in nutrition. When they consume a lot of milk and wheat products, stomach acid can cause stomach cancer. In the evening, if they eat rice, bread, bulgur and liver, they cannot digest. In the evening, they can consume vegetable food, meat, fish, salads. White cabbage and cauliflower make awesome gas. They can eat sauerkraut. Broccoli and Brussels sprouts are very good for them. Those who have zero blood group may be healthy by increasing the meat. If they do not, they complain of heartburn and helicobacter infection. Finally, people with a blood group of 0 who love to consume dairy products have stones, sand or lime in their kidney.

<u>**BLOOD GROUP O**</u>

<u>Beneficial Foods (At the same time, the safest drugs) :</u>

* Meat Products: Beef, beef, mutton and wild animal (may be a little oily); the fish; fresh village eggs.

* Oils: Olive oil, flax oil, walnut oil, animal oils (tallow / tail oil).

* Vegetables: Artichoke, kale, broccoli, chicory, lettuce, spinach, arugula, parsley, chard, every green leafy vegetable, radish (especially horseradish), beetroot, onion, garlic, zucchini, pumpkin.

* Fruits: Fig, grape (especially black grape), plum, plum plum, cherry, cherry, grapefruit and juice, black mulberry, watermelon, mango.

* Spices: Red chili peppers, ginger, saffron, carob, turmeric, cumin, coriander, flax seed.

* Teas: Rosehip, marjoram, linden, green tea, thyme, tarragon, rosemary, hawthorn, olive leaf, rosecot.

* Others: Genuine honey and natural mineral water.

* Nuts: Walnuts, unroasted pumpkin seeds.

Edible Foods :

* **Meat Products:** Chicken, turkey and wild bird meat.

* **Dairy Products:** Naturally produced butter, cream (occasionally), homemade yogurt, homemade kefir, naturally produced cottage cheese, sheep and goats cheese, old cheddar, leather bottle cheese - these can be eaten 1-3 times a week; sheep, goat, camel milk (cow milk can only be consumed in dairy desserts, with cinnamon and ginger.)

* **Vegetables-Fruits:** All kinds of raw cabbage (except gas-producing in the intestines); Jerusalem artichoke, black eyed peas, kidney beans, green beans, chickpea, eggplant, celery, tangerine and any fruit, vegetable and food that are not in the category of harmful.

* **Cereals :** Rice and its products, buckwheat and its varieties, rye and its varieties, starch wheat (old Turkish wheat) varieties; domestic corn and maize products.

* **Nuts:** Sesame and its products (make sure that tahini is not mixed with sunflower oil), walnuts, unroastedor newly roasted pine nuts, hazelnuts, almonds and almond oil, chestnuts.

<u>**Harmful Foods :**</u>

Milk and dairy products (except " edible ones "), wheat and wheat products, peanuts, cauliflower, oranges, aloe vera, tomato paste, coffee, black tea, foods and drinks that form gas in the stomach and intestines.

NOTE: Healthy people may consume foods and beverages in the category of harmful foods occasionally (not during recovery) if they are natural and not genetically modified.

<u>**Harmful Foods For Everyone :**</u>

Ready-made ice cream, genetically modified wheat and its products (especially type 405-550), genetically modified corn and its products, genetically modified American soybean, refined and hydrogenated oils, margarines, roasted, and dried drynuts, ketchup, chemical vinegars (white vinegar spirit products), stale foods, pre-cooked and reheated foods, chewing gum, ready-made food and beverages, sweeteners, genetically modified wheat and corn starch, glucose, fructose,doped market olives, doped ready pickles. All kinds of factory processed packaged products (teas, tomato paste, olives).

" (Blood Group A)

Now, we'll talk about the nutrition of the blood group A . In blood group nutrition, the most problematic stomachs are those with group 0 and A. Especially those with blood type A always have digestion problems because they eat meat even though stomach acids are produced less. Meat-eating blood type A is in a very difficult situation. But when he quits meat, his stomachs return to normal immediately. Blood type A should consume meat once a week at most. But blood type A can carry zero (A0). Then the blood group may have the properties of zero. Sometimes the adjectives of blood group zero are dominant in those with blood group A.

 "Then we tell them to reproduce and consume meat twice a week," says Doctor Aidin SALIH [1]. Aidin SALIH [1], " When someone with blood type A arrives, I ask him how many tooth fillings he has because if he has a tooth filling in the mouth, that person will carry zero group blood. " says. She also says, " When I ask if their parents' blood group is zero, they say 'yes' and they are surprised that I know this."

Mehmet Ali BULUT [2], in his book, says the followings for the blood group A: "They have a delicate and light digestive system. If we go on from the car sample where we compare the digestive systems to the engine, we can compare the engine of the people in the group A to that of a vehicle working with 'unleaded gasoline'. Super gasoline (white meat and dairy products) can even harm it. Besides, it is worse for them to use diesel (red meat) and diesel (beef and similar hard-to-digest food) ... Doctors encourage people to avoid red meat, fat, salt, sugar and bread after a certain age, this is both true and false. It is true, yes; because A groups should definitely stay away from red meat. Group O should avoid bread, Group B should avoid lentils and chicken, AB group should avoid oil and all groups should avoid salt and sugar after a certain age."

The main diseases encountered by those with blood group A are: Swelling of the stomach, belching, vomiting, anemia, elephant disease and cancer. Since stomach acid is produced less, they experience bloating. That's why they can't digest red meat. In them, heavy metabolic wastes are formed due to meat and cause sedation or inflammatory rheumatism. Mixed food or meat dishes will rot without indigestion. It creates gas as it decays. Then burping occurs with gas. Aidin SALIH ' says at one of her conferences: "His doctor said to someone who had previously had reflux surgery: - You will never have reflux anymore, you will not even burp." And again, she says, " Well, how will he not burp? Even, if this patient is blood type A, he will crack and burst. Because even a small mistake, gas is formed immediately."

Those with blood type A digest wheat products very well. Metabolic waste of wheat products does not accumulate in the feet, only bad fats accumulate. The most severe elephant disease occurs in those with blood type A because it is not possible to remove and melt those fats in any way. Wheat is the best food for those with blood type A. They eat rice, bulgur and everything with bread. They are those who eat bread with bread. If they do not eat bread, they will starve. Let them consume bread other than white bread. Even if they do not eat fruit, they will be healthy.

<u>BLOOD GROUP A</u>

<u>Beneficial Foods (At the same time, the safest drugs) :</u>

* **Meat Products:** Fish: cod, carp, sardine, mackerel, red perch.

* **Oils:** Olive oil, walnut oil, almond oil, tail oil-tallow oil.

* **Vegetables:** Black eyed peas beans, soy and its products (soy natural, genetically unaltered), artichoke, chicory, lettuce, carrot and carrot juice, beetroot and juice, purslane and juice, zucchini, leek, spinach, chard, white cabbage, broccoli, Jerusalem artichoke , garlic, onion, celery, parsley and all kinds of green leafy vegetables.

* **Fruits:** Apricot, berry, fig, grape, cherry, plum, grapefruit, lemon, damson.

* **Spices:** Ginger, turmeric, cardamom (cardamone), mustard weed, flaxseed, cumin, thyme, rosemary, naturally grown aloe vera, magnesium sulfate (English salt), clove, cassia.

* **Teas:** Rosehip, fresh roasted coffee, green tea, rosemary, linden.

* **Others:** Boiled grape juice.

BLOOD GROUP A

Beneficial Foods (Continuing) :

* **Dairy Products:** Kefir and kefir juice; yoghurt and yoghurt juice.

* **Carbohydrates:** Wheat products and bread (amarant or old Turkish wheat), rye products and bread, oat products and bread, buckwheat products.

* **Legumes:** All kinds of lentils, haricot beans (pearl beans), chickpeas.

* **Nuts:** Peanuts, walnuts, pumpkin seeds, bitter almonds, almonds.

BLOOD GROUP A

Edible Foods:

* **Meat Products:** *Chicken and turkey meat (sheep-lamb meat can be eaten once during sacrifice feasts or once every 10 - 14 days), fresh eggs.*

* **Dairy Products:** *Sheep, goat cheese and milk, feta cheese, pickled cheese, old cheese, leather bottle cheese, mozzarella; camel, sheep milk. (Attention should be paid to the milk and yeast of cheese.)*

* **Others:** *Honey, unrefined sugar, chestnut, sesame and its products, rice and its products, corn and its products (domestic corn, not genetically modified American corn), barley varieties, red beans, radish, pomegranate and fruit, vegetables and foods that are not included in the harmful group.*

NOTE: In groups with blood group A and carrying O, (AO) red meat can be consumed once a week. A who do not carry O can consume (AA) red meat only once every two weeks or once a month. While honey is not recommended for AA groups,

AO grpups may occasionally use honey.

<u>**BLOOD GROUP A**</u>

<u>*Harmful Foods :*</u>

Every meat (except chicken and turkey), sea animals (crayfish, squid etc.) and caviar, cow's milk, butter and any oil or fat (excluding fish oil, veal oil, olive oil and flax oil), potatoes, chili peppers, tomato, tomato paste, black tea, tangerine, orange and juice, mineral water.

NOTE: Healthy people may consume foods and beverages in the category of harmful foods occasionally (not during recovery) if they are natural and not genetically modified.

<u>*Harmful Foods For Everyone :*</u>

Ready-made ice cream, genetically modified wheat and its products (especially type 405-550), genetically modified corn and its products, genetically modified American soybean, refined and hydrogenated oils, margarines, roasted, and dried drynuts, ketchup, chemical vinegars (white vinegar spirit products), stale foods, pre-cooked and reheated foods, chewing gum, ready-made food and beverages, sweeteners, genetically modified wheat and corn starch, glucose, fructose,doped market olives, doped ready pickles. All kinds of factory processed packaged products (teas, tomato paste, olives).

Now, we will talk mainly about B blood group nutrition. If a person's little toe is curled and hidden inward, his blood type is B. Even if the blood group is B, if the little toe is normal, that person is carrying O. In this case, O of the blood group B's predominate. Already, blood groups B and O are very similar. If the blood group B carries O, his temper is also docile. However, those with blood type BB are not like that.

Blood type B is a very interesting blood type. Those with blood group B can be both BB and BO. Therefore, there are those among blood group B's that look like blood group O. People with blood group B are the people who have weakest kidneys and urinary systems. The kidney capacity is low in all B's except blood group BO. Those with blood group B will have a large upper jaw. If it is narrow, he definitely carries O. The part we call the upper jaw is the place from the nose to the upper lip level. The nail on the little finger of those with BB will be very short. It is also due to kidneys. Since the kidneys of those with blood group B are sensitive and their capacity is low; they are prone to excessive sweating, headache, blood pressure, diabetes and cholesterol imbalance.

Mehmet Ali BULUT [2], in his book, says the following for the blood group B: "The digestive systems have strong enzymes. In the phrase, even if the acids of the B groups are dropped on the stone, they dissolve it. If we need to liken their digestive mechanism to the engine, engines that use fuel-oil for B's category are probably the best examples. There is research results that Turks are the main blood group in the period of nomadic life. It is important for those in group B to get up before sunrise. Sleeping at sunrise does not disturb any group as much as those from group B. Sheep, lamb, goat, rabbit and wild meat (venison) is healing,   not only food but also medicine for groups B." Dr. Aidin SALIH [1] says for those with blood group B: "Because their kidneys are weak, they are very prone to skin diseases. Because the skin is the second kidney. Therefore, excessive sweating appears first, and then eczema and psoriasis are seen. Skin diseases are the salvation of blood type B, as their kidneys are weak. Because metabolic waste is discharged through the skin. Of course, a general treatment, not regional, should be given to psoriasis. For blood group B, diabetes, blood pressure, and cholesterol imbalance and thyroid problems are very natural. Because when the kidneys are weak, the adrenal gland weakens over time. "

Those with blood group B are prone to mental problems. They are also prone to violence, but this is not due to thyroid. The path of energy crosses the head, going down to the eyebrows, thus affecting the brain. Headache is a neurological problem, as the brain is affected and headaches are very severe, and water circulation is disturbed. It is normal for them to have headaches on full moon and new moon days (6 days a month). Because the moon draws the water of the world at this time. Humans also consist of 70% water and 30% substance.

<u>BLOOD GROUP B</u>

<u>Beneficial Foods (At the same time, the safest drugs) :</u>

* **Meat Products:** Sheep, lamb, goat, turkey, rabbit and wild meat, trout, sardine, red sea bass, whiting, cod, caviar, bey fish, fresh egg.

* **Oils:** Olive oil, tallow / tail oil

* **Vegetables:** Eggplant, celery, beetroot, carrot, all kinds of cabbage, cauliflower, potato, all peppers, dandelion, parsley and all kinds of greens.

* **Fruits:** Plum, watermelon, banana, grape, fig, cherry, cherry, currant, peach, citrus (tangerine, orange, grapefruit, lemon)

* **Spices:** Cumin, fenugreek, chili, curry, basil (basil), magnesium sulfate (English salt), coriander.

* **Dairy Products:** Yogurt, natural milk, natural feta cheese, old cheddar cheese, mozzarella, sheep and goat milk and cheese.

* **Others:** Genuine honey, boiled grape juice.

<u>Beneficial Foods (Continuing) :</u>

* Teas: Chamomile, thyme, lavender, cockroach, mint, green tea.

* Legumes: Green lentils.

* Carbohydrates: Oats and varieties, rice and varieties, natural wheat and varieties.

* Nuts: Walnuts.

BLOOD GROUP B

Edible Foods:

* Meat Products: Each meat (excluding chicken and goose).

* Dairy Products: Butter, cream.

* Carbohydrates: Barley and its products.

* Legumes: Kidney beans, white beans, pearl beans, green beans.

* Teas: Untreated tea, fresh coffee.

* Nuts: Sweet almonds.

* Vegetables, fruits : Mushrooms, zucchini, any fruits and vegetables that do not fit in "Harmful" groups, chestnuts.

* Spices: Cassia, goat horn, mint, anise, cocoa, sugar candy, flaxseed, thyme.

BLOOD GROUP B

<u>**Harmful Foods :**</u>

Sea animals, chicken and goose meat, every lentil, chickpeas, peanuts, Pistachios, sunflower seeds, sesame and its products, corn and its products, rye and its products, black wheat and its products, artichoke, aloe vera, coconut, every oil (excluding olive oil, flax oil), black pepper, white pepper, tomato paste, soy sauce, cinnamon.

NOTE: Healthy people may consume foods and beverages in the category of harmful foods occasionally (not during recovery) if they are natural and not genetically modified.

<u>**Harmful Foods For Everyone :**</u>

Ready-made ice cream, genetically modified wheat and its products (especially type 405-550), genetically modified corn and its products, genetically modified American soybean, refined and hydrogenated oils, margarines, roasted, and dried drynuts, ketchup, chemical vinegars (white vinegar spirit products), stale foods, pre-cooked and reheated foods, chewing gum, ready-made food and beverages, sweeteners, genetically modified wheat and corn starch, glucose, fructose,doped market olives, doped ready pickles. All kinds of factory processed packaged products (teas, tomato paste, olives).

* (Blood Group AB)

Now, we will talk mainly about nutrition in blood group AB. Dr. Aidin SALIH ¹ said at her conference, which she talked about blood groups: " The situation is somewhat complicated in those with blood group AB. Both A's and B's can be dominant in this blood group. The condition of those with blood type AB depends on whether A or B is more dominant. How do you notice this? When taking a blood group test, if clotting is earlier in B, this means B is dominant. If A coagulates earlier, this means A is more dominant. Those with blood group AB should ask for this when taking a test. Thus it is clearly known which one is more dominant and diet can be made accordingly. This situation is not understood in hijama. If the person with blood type AB can vomit easily, make sure that A is more dominant in him. But if he can't vomit, B is more dominant. Because those with blood group O and B do not vomit at all, except for special cases and diseases. The blood type most sensitive to fat is AB. The most beneficial oil for those in the AB blood group is undoubtedly olive oil as for all other groups. Olive oil is one of the suitable fuels suitable for human nature. Then comes walnut oil. Fats harmful to the AB blood group are;

avocado and sunflower oil, coconut oil, corn oil, cottonseed oil, sesame oil and peanut oil. "

In his book, Mehmet Ali BULUT [2] says the following for the blood group AB: " Blood group AB refers to hybridity. I liken the engine structure of those in the AB group to the engine running on 'super petrol'. AB's digestive system is slightly more sensitive than A's. However, they are slightly better than A's in red meat consumption because ABs are somewhat like B. While consumption of red meat is very limited in group A, ABs can easily eat mutton / lamb meat. Turkey meat is under the category of 'healing' for the blood group AB. "

"The weakest immune system group," says Dr. Aidin SALIH [1] for the blood group AB. She continues her speech as follows: "That is why they are the most susceptible to cancer. You will see that almost 60% -70% of cancer patients are AB. Then A, then B, and finally O." In M. Ali Bulut's [2] book it is written that "harmful food consumption is illness" for the AB group. If digestion is impaired, toxic residue is formed. Liver diseases occur. They need to swallow garlic. They shall research. Apply 21 days of garlic cure, 1-2 times a year. They shall increase the green vegetables. They need to drink quality water.

BLOOD GROUP AB

Beneficial Foods (At the same time, the safest drugs) :

* Meat Products: Mutton, rabbit and turkey meat, fish; red perch, sardine, cod, beyfish, fresh egg.

* Oils: Olive oil, walnut oil and tallow, tail oil.

* Vegetables: Cucumber, cauliflower, white cabbage, eggplant, beetroot, purslane, spinach, collard greens, lettuce, carrot, chard, broccoli, garlic, onion, celery, parsley and all green leafy vegetables, sea kale (laminaria)

* Fruits: Fig, grape, cherry, cherry, plum, grapefruit, lemon, plum plum, watermelon, pineapple.

* Spices: Ginger, cumin, turmeric, coriander, fenugreek, cardamom (cardamon), flaxseed.

* Teas: Rosehip, chamomile, green tea, thyme, lavender, nettle, fresh coffee.

* Others: Halis honey, molasses, magnesium sulfate (English salt).

* Legumes: Green lentils.

BLOOD GROUP AB

Beneficial Foods (Continuing) :

* Carbohydrates: Buckwheat products and bread, oat products and bread, rice products and bread, soft wheat (old turkish wheat) products and bread, barley products and bread.

* Dairy Products: Yoghurt, natural feta cheese, old cheddar, goat and sheep milk and cheese.

* Nuts: Peanuts, walnuts, almonds, hazelnuts.

<u>BLOOD GROUP AB</u>

<u>Edible Foods:</u>

* **Meat Products:** Caviar, occasionally beef / beef.

* **Dairy Products:** Single cow's milk, occasionally butter.

* **Legumes:** Kidney beans, white beans.

* **Nuts:** Pistachio.

* **Vegetables, fruits :** Leeks, tomatoes, apricots, mulberries, melons and foods that are not included in "Harmful" group , fruits and vegetables, pomegranate and its juice, banana, tangerine, chestnut.

* **Spices:** Thyme, mint, unrefined sugar.

NOTE: It is difficult to talk about the list of benefits-pests with strict rules for the blood group AB. B-weighted ABs can change their nutrition programs according to group B and A-weighted ABs can change their diet according to group A. The AB group must be attentive so that the people of this group can decide what is harmful and what is good.

BLOOD GROUP AB

Harmful Foods :

Chicken meat, sea animals, corn and its products, chickpeas, rye bread, sesame and its products, cowpea beans, sunflower beans, chili peppers, black and white pepper, tomato paste, orange and juice, avocado, artichoke, radish, aloe vera and any oil or fat (excluding olive oil and walnut oil), orange, coconut.

NOTE: Healthy people may consume foods and beverages in the category of harmful foods occasionally (not during recovery) if they are natural and not genetically modified.

Harmful Foods For Everyone :

Ready-made ice cream, genetically modified wheat and its products (especially type 405-550), genetically modified corn and its products, genetically modified American soybean, refined and hydrogenated oils, margarines, roasted, and dried drynuts, ketchup, chemical vinegars (white vinegar spirit products), stale foods, pre-cooked and reheated foods, chewing gum, ready-made food and beverages, sweeteners, genetically modified wheat and corn starch, glucose, fructose,doped market olives, doped ready pickles. All kinds of factory processed packaged products (teas, tomato paste, olives).

TRANSLATED AND COMPILED BY CEYHUN EMANET (PRONUNCIATION IN ENGLISH: JAYHOON EMANETT)

✖✖✖

WE WISH EVERYONE HEALTH, GOODNESS AND WELL-BEING FROM ALLAH

✖✖✖

REFERENCES:

1) Aidin SALIH

Book : Son Söz /Gerçek Tıp Dersleri Cilt 1 (Final Word / Real Medical Lessons Volume 1)

2) Mehmet Ali BULUT

Book : Can Boğazdan Çıkar (Life Comes out of the Throat.)